MW01170342

The Complete Guide To An
Effective Antiviral Medication For
The Treatment Of Viral Skin
Infections, Herpes Simplex Virus
(Hsv), Genital Herps, Cold Sores
And Other Conditions

Dr. David Krishna

1

Table of Contents

CHAPTER ONE 4

ACYCLOVIR CREAM GUIDE 4

REASON AND UTILIZATION OF ACYCLOVIR CREAM 5

SIGNS AND USES 9

CHAPTER TWO 15

CONDITIONS TREATED BY ACYCLOVIR CREAM 15

THE MOST EFFECTIVE METHOD TO UTILIZE ACYCLOVIR CREAM 21

CHAPTER THREE...26

DOSAGE AND ADMINISTRATION 26

POSSIBLE INCIDENTAL EFFECTS 30

UNCOMMON HOWEVER SERIOUS AFTEREFFECTS..32

CHAPTER FOUR 36

NORMAL INCIDENTAL EFFECTS....................36

SERIOUS INCIDENTAL EFFECTS (INTERESTING HOWEVER EXTREME)..................................39

ALLERGIC REACTIONS RESPONSES AND WHAT TO DO...43

CHAPTER FIVE 50

COLLABORATIONS WITH DIFFERENT DRUGS
....50

WELLBEING AND SAFEGUARDS....................54

OUTLINE AND IMPORTANT POINTS ABOUT
ACYCLOVIR CREAM 61

CONCLUSION...63

THE END...66

CHAPTER ONE

ACYCLOVIR CREAM GUIDE

Acyclovir cream is a skin antiviral prescription used to treat specific viral skin diseases brought about by the herpes simplex infection (HSV). It is normally recommended to oversee conditions like mouth blisters (herpes labialis) and genital herpes (outside injuries). The cream contains acyclovir as its dynamic fixing, which decreases the seriousness and term of side effects related with these viral diseases.

REASON AND UTILIZATION OF ACYCLOVIR CREAM

The motivation behind acyclovir cream is to give confined treatment to specific viral skin contaminations brought about by the herpes simplex infection (HSV). The cream contains acyclovir as its dynamic fixing, which is an antiviral drug successful against herpes infections. Acyclovir cream is principally utilized for the accompanying purposes:

* Mouth blisters (Herpes Labialis):

Acyclovir cream is generally used to treat mouth blisters, otherwise called herpes labialis, which are little, agonizing rankles or injuries that show up close by the lips and mouth. Mouth blisters are brought about by HSV-1 (herpes simplex infection type 1) and are exceptionally infectious. Acyclovir cream decreases the seriousness of side effects, like torment, tingling, and redness, and speeds up the recuperating system of the mouth blisters.

* Genital Herpes (Outside Sores):

In instances of genital herpes brought about by HSV-2 (herpes simplex infection type 2), acyclovir cream can be utilized to treat the outside sores on the genital and butt-centric regions. It mitigates side effects, like torment, uneasiness, and tingling, and advances quicker recuperating of the injuries.

* Other Confined Herpes Contaminations:

Acyclovir cream may likewise be utilized to treat other confined herpes contaminations brought about by HSV-1 or HSV-2, for example, herpes gladiatorum (herpes disease among competitors), herpes whitlow (disease of the fingers), and herpes simplex keratitis (eye contamination).

Acyclovir cream is a skin detailing, meaning it is applied straightforwardly to the impacted region of the skin. At the point when applied right on time during the beginning of side effects, the cream can be best in lessening the seriousness and term of the viral contamination. It doesn't fix herpes contaminations however deals with the side effects and speeds up the recuperating system.

It's fundamental to follow the suggested measurement and application guidelines given by a medical care proficient or as shown on the cream's bundling.

The cream ought to simply be applied to the impacted outside skin surfaces and ought not be utilized inside the mouth, eyes, or vagina.

SIGNS AND USES

Acyclovir is an antiviral prescription used to treat viral diseases brought about by the herpes simplex infection (HSV) and the varicella-zoster infection (VZV). The principal signs and uses of acyclovir include:

* Treatment of Herpes Simplex Infection (HSV) Contaminations:

Mouth blisters (Herpes Labialis): Acyclovir is regularly used to treat mouth blisters that show up close by the lips and mouth. These mouth blisters are brought about by HSV-1 (herpes simplex infection type 1). Acyclovir cream is frequently applied topically to the impacted region to diminish side effects and advance quicker recuperating.

* Genital Herpes: Acyclovir is utilized to treat genital herpes, which is brought about by HSV-2 (herpes simplex infection type 2). It lightens side effects, like difficult genital wounds, tingling, and uneasiness.

* Herpes Gladiatorum: This alludes to a herpes disease normal among competitors engaged with physical games. Acyclovir might be utilized to deal with the skin sores related with this condition.

* Herpes Whitlow: Acyclovir might be endorsed to treat herpetic whitlow, which is a herpes disease influencing the fingers.

* Herpes Simplex Keratitis: Acyclovir balm or eye drops are utilized to treat herpes simplex keratitis, a disease influencing the eyes.

* Treatment of Varicella-Zoster Infection (VZV) Diseases:

Chickenpox (Varicella): Acyclovir might be utilized to treat serious instances of chickenpox in specific populaces, like immunocompromised people or grown-ups.

* Shingles (Herpes Zoster): Acyclovir is utilized to treat shingles, a difficult rash brought about by the reactivation of the varicella-zoster infection in people who have had chickenpox before.

* Prophylaxis (Preventive Treatment): Acyclovir might be utilized as prophylaxis in people at high gamble of extreme herpes infection diseases, like those going

through organ transplantation or people with compromised resistant frameworks.

It's essential to take note of that while acyclovir can help oversee and lighten side effects of herpes and varicella-zoster infection contaminations, it's anything but a fix. Once tainted with these infections, they stay in the body in a torpid state and can reactivate, causing repetitive diseases. Acyclovir assists with lessening the seriousness and span of dynamic flare-ups and forestall confusions yet doesn't wipe out the infection from the body.

The particular measurements and term of acyclovir therapy rely upon the singular's condition, clinical history, and safe status. Continuously adhere to the guidelines given by your medical services supplier or as shown on the medicine's bundling for protected and viable use. In the event that you suspect you have a herpes or varicella-zoster infection contamination or experience any connected side effects, look for clinical guidance for legitimate determination and fitting treatment.

CHAPTER TWO

CONDITIONS TREATED BY ACYCLOVIR CREAM

Acyclovir cream is essentially used to treat viral skin diseases brought about by the herpes simplex infection (HSV), explicitly HSV-1 (herpes simplex infection type 1) and HSV-2 (herpes simplex infection type 2). The cream is applied topically to the impacted region and is viable in dealing with the accompanying circumstances:

* Mouth blisters (Herpes Labialis):

Mouth blisters, otherwise called fever rankles, are little, difficult liquid filled rankles or injuries that normally show up close by the lips, mouth, and now and again the nose. They are brought about by HSV-1, and the underlying disease is many times gained during adolescence. Mouth blisters can be set off by different elements, like openness to daylight, stress, or a debilitated resistant framework. Acyclovir cream can assist with decreasing the seriousness and span of mouth blisters and give help from side effects like agony, tingling, and redness.

* Genital Herpes (Outside Sores):

Genital herpes is a physically sent contamination brought about by

HSV-2. It can cause excruciating and bothersome bruises or ulcers on the genital and butt-centric regions. Acyclovir cream can be utilized to treat the outer injuries and assist with lightening uneasiness and advance quicker recuperating. In any case, it is crucial for note that acyclovir cream isn't a solution for genital herpes, and it doesn't forestall the transmission of the infection to sexual accomplices.

* Other Restricted Herpes Contaminations:

Acyclovir cream may likewise be utilized to treat other restricted herpes contaminations brought about by HSV-1 or HSV-2. These include:

* Herpes Gladiatorum: This alludes to a herpes disease normal among competitors engaged with physical games, like wrestling. Acyclovir cream can be applied to the impacted skin sores to assist with dealing with the condition.

* Herpes Whitlow: Herpetic whitlow is a herpes contamination that influences the fingers. Acyclovir cream might be utilized to treat the bruises on the fingers and decrease inconvenience.

* Herpes Simplex Keratitis: Acyclovir salve or eye drops are utilized to treat herpes simplex keratitis, which is a viral contamination influencing the eyes' cornea.

* It's critical to utilize acyclovir cream as coordinated by a medical care proficient and to begin therapy at the earliest indications of a flare-up. Applying the cream right off the bat throughout the contamination can prompt improved results in lessening side effects and advancing mending. Furthermore, acyclovir cream is best when utilized during the

dynamic period of the viral disease and not as a preventive measure.

On the off chance that you suspect you have any of these herpes diseases or experience side effects like mouth blisters or genital sores, counsel a medical services supplier for legitimate conclusion and direction on the utilization of acyclovir cream. They can survey your condition and decide whether acyclovir cream is a proper treatment choice for your particular case.

THE MOST EFFECTIVE METHOD TO UTILIZE ACYCLOVIR CREAM

Utilizing acyclovir cream appropriately is fundamental to guarantee its adequacy in treating viral skin contaminations brought about by the herpes simplex infection (HSV). Here are basic principles on the most proficient method to utilize acyclovir cream:

* Wash Hands: Prior to applying acyclovir cream, clean up completely with cleanser and water to guarantee that the impacted region stays clean and to forestall the spread of disease.

* Clean the Impacted Region: Delicately clean the impacted skin with gentle cleanser and water. Wipe the region off with a spotless towel or permit it to air dry prior to applying the cream.

* Utilization of Acyclovir Cream:

Crush a modest quantity of acyclovir cream (generally a ½ inch or less) onto at the tip of your finger or a q-tip. Utilize sufficient cream to cover the whole mouth blister, genital injury, or impacted region.

Cautiously and equitably apply the cream to the impacted region. Try not to get the cream in your eyes, mouth, or inside the vagina or rear-end. Assuming inadvertent contact happens, wash completely with water.

Tenderly rub the cream into the skin until it is consumed.

* Recurrence of Use: Acyclovir cream is commonly applied 5 times each day, about at regular intervals, during waking hours. Adhere to your medical care supplier's directions or the rules on the cream's bundling in regards to the particular dosing plan for your condition.

* Span of Treatment: Keep utilizing acyclovir cream for the

full endorsed course, regardless of whether the side effects improve or vanish before the treatment is finished. Finishing the full tasks of treatment is fundamental to guarantee the best outcomes and forestall repeat.

* Safeguards: Try not to contact the mouth blister or impacted region pointlessly to decrease the gamble of spreading the infection to different pieces of your body or to others.

Clean up in the wake of applying the cream to keep away from unintentional contact with different region of the body or others.

Assuming you wear contact focal points, eliminate them prior to applying acyclovir cream to the region around the eyes. Stand by somewhere around 15 minutes in the wake of applying the cream prior to reinserting the focal points.

Try not to apply wraps or dressings over the cream except if trained to do as such by your medical services supplier.

CHAPTER THREE

DOSAGE AND ADMINISTRATION

The measurement and organization of acyclovir cream rely upon the particular condition being dealt with and the medical care supplier's proposals. The following are common rules for the measurements and organization of acyclovir cream for various signs:

* Mouth blisters (Herpes Labialis):

For grown-ups and kids 12 years old and more seasoned: Apply a slender layer of acyclovir cream to the impacted region on the lips or face like clockwork, five times each day, for a sum of five days.

* Genital Herpes (Outer Injuries):

For grown-ups and youngsters 12 years old and more seasoned: Apply an adequate measure of acyclovir cream to cover the genital or butt-centric injuries like clockwork, five times each day, for a sum of five days.

* Other Restricted Herpes Diseases (e.g., Herpes Gladiatorum, Herpes Whitlow, Herpes Simplex Keratitis):

The measurement and treatment span for other limited herpes contaminations might change relying upon the seriousness and explicit condition. Adhere to your medical services supplier's directions for the fitting dosing and length.

* General Organization Rules:

Clean up when applying acyclovir cream to forestall the spread of the infection and guarantee tidiness.

Clean the impacted region with gentle cleanser and water, and wipe it off prior to applying the cream.

Apply the cream delicately and equitably to the impacted region. Try not to get the cream in your eyes, mouth, or mucous films.

Utilize sufficient cream to cover the whole mouth blister, genital injury, or impacted skin region.

It's vital to begin utilizing acyclovir cream as quickly as time permits after the primary indications of a mouth blister or genital sore show up. Early application can prompt improved results in lessening side effects and advancing mending.

Assuming you are utilizing other skin prescriptions or treatments on a similar region, counsel your medical care supplier or drug specialist to guarantee there are no expected communications.

For people with compromised kidney capability or other ailments, measurement changes might be vital. Continuously follow your medical care supplier's suggestions and don't surpass the recommended portion.

POSSIBLE INCIDENTAL EFFECTS

Acyclovir, similar to any medicine, may cause secondary effects in certain people. Not every person encounter aftereffect, and their seriousness can differ from one individual to another. The most well-known results of acyclovir are normally gentle and include:

* Skin Bothering: A few people might encounter gentle skin disturbance at the application site while utilizing acyclovir cream. This can incorporate redness, tingling, or a consuming sensation.

* Dry or Stripping Skin: now and again, acyclovir cream might make the skin become dry or strip at the application site.

* Cerebral pain: Certain individuals might encounter migraines while utilizing acyclovir,

albeit this incidental effect is somewhat interesting.

These incidental effects are typically transitory and ought to determine all alone as your body acclimates to the prescription. Nonetheless, assuming these incidental effects persevere or become vexatious, contact your medical services supplier or drug specialist for direction.

UNCOMMON HOWEVER SERIOUS AFTEREFFECTS

While uncommon, acyclovir can cause more serious secondary effects in certain people. In the event that you experience any of the accompanying side effects, look for guaranteed clinical consideration:

* Unfavorably susceptible Responses: Indications of a hypersensitive response might incorporate hives, tingling, enlarging of the face, lips, tongue, or throat, extreme tipsiness, or trouble relaxing.

* Extreme Skin Responses: Once in a blue moon, acyclovir might cause extreme skin responses, for example, Stevens-Johnson disorder or harmful epidermal necrolysis, which are serious and possibly dangerous circumstances. Side effects might incorporate

rankling, stripping, or a rash that covers a huge region of the body.

* Neurological Side effects: In uncommon cases, acyclovir might cause neurological side effects like disarray, mental trips, unsettling, seizures, or trouble talking.

* Assuming you experience any of these extreme incidental effects, quit utilizing acyclovir right away and look for crisis clinical consideration.

* It's fundamental to illuminate your medical services supplier about any known sensitivities, ailments, or prescriptions you are taking prior to beginning acyclovir

therapy. Your medical care supplier can survey your singular gamble factors and screen you for any expected incidental effects during therapy.

CHAPTER FOUR

NORMAL INCIDENTAL EFFECTS

Normal symptoms of acyclovir are generally gentle and may include:

* Skin Bothering: The most well-known symptom of acyclovir cream is gentle skin aggravation at the application site. This can appear as redness, tingling, or a consuming sensation.

* Dry or Stripping Skin: A few people might encounter dryness or stripping of the skin at the site where the cream is applied.

* Migraine: at times, people might encounter cerebral pains while utilizing acyclovir cream, albeit this secondary effect is generally interesting.

* It's critical to take note of that these normal incidental effects are by and large brief and will generally determine all alone as your body changes with the drug. Assuming you experience any of these aftereffects and think that they are annoying, counsel your medical care supplier or drug specialist for guidance on the best way to oversee them.

The vast majority endure acyclovir cream well without encountering huge aftereffects. Be that as it may, individual reactions to drugs can change, and a few people might be more delicate to specific parts of the cream.

Assuming that you have any worries about the incidental affects you are encountering or are uncertain assuming that they are connected with acyclovir cream, go ahead and out to your medical care supplier. They can give direction and decide if any changes are essential for your treatment.

SERIOUS INCIDENTAL EFFECTS (INTERESTING HOWEVER EXTREME)

While serious symptoms of acyclovir are uncommon, they can happen in certain people. Assuming you experience any of the accompanying extreme incidental effects, look for sure fire clinical consideration or contact your medical services supplier:

* Hypersensitive Responses: Certain individuals might have an unfavorably susceptible response

39

to acyclovir. Side effects of an unfavorably susceptible response can include:

* Hives or rash

* Tingling or enlarging, particularly of the face, lips, tongue, or throat

* Serious wooziness or unsteadiness

* Trouble breathing or snugness in the chest

* Serious Skin Responses: Once in a while, acyclovir might cause extreme skin responses, like

Stevens-Johnson disorder or poisonous epidermal necrolysis. These are serious and possibly perilous circumstances described by boundless skin rankling, stripping, and injuries. Assuming you experience any strange skin changes, rashes, or rankles, look for sure fire clinical consideration.

* Neurological Side effects: In uncommon cases, acyclovir might prompt neurological aftereffects. Assuming you experience any of the accompanying side effects, look for clinical consideration:

* Disarray or confusion

* Pipedreams or unusual way of behaving

* Seizures or spasms

* Trouble talking or slurred discourse

* Kidney Issues: Albeit phenomenal, acyclovir can influence kidney capability in certain people. Indications of kidney issues might remember changes for pee recurrence, dim hued pee, or expanding in the hands, feet, or lower legs. In the event that you experience any kidney-related side effects, contact your medical services supplier.

Recall that serious secondary effects with acyclovir are interesting, and most people endure the medicine well without encountering extreme unfriendly responses. It's fundamental to adhere to your medical services supplier's guidelines with respect to the legitimate use and measurement of acyclovir.

In the event that you have a known history of sensitivities or have encountered serious secondary effects with acyclovir or comparable prescriptions previously, illuminate your medical care supplier prior to beginning the therapy.

ALLERGIC REACTIONS RESPONSES AND WHAT TO DO

Hypersensitive responses to acyclovir are generally uncommon yet can happen in certain people. In the event that you experience indications of a hypersensitive response in the wake of utilizing acyclovir or some other prescription, it's crucial for make a prompt move to guarantee your security and prosperity. Hypersensitive responses can go from gentle to serious and might possibly life-compromise. This is what to do assuming you suspect you are having a hypersensitive response to acyclovir:

* Perceive the Side effects: Hypersensitive responses can appear in different ways. Normal indications of an unfavorably susceptible response might include:

* Hives or rash: Irritated, raised red welts on the skin.

* Tingling: Summed up or centered tingling, particularly on the skin or around the mouth.

Enlarging: Expanding of the face, lips, tongue, throat, or other body parts.

* Trouble Relaxing: Windedness, wheezing, or a sensation of snugness in the chest.

* Unsteadiness or Discombobulation: Feeling weak or mixed up.

* Queasiness or Retching: Feeling debilitated to your stomach or heaving.

* Quit Utilizing Acyclovir: On the off chance that you suspect an unfavorably susceptible response to acyclovir, quit utilizing the drug right away. Suspend the cream or some other acyclovir item you are utilizing.

* Look for Crisis Clinical Assistance: In the event that you experience extreme side effects, for example, trouble breathing, enlarging of the face or throat, or any indications of hypersensitivity (a serious and possibly hazardous unfavorably susceptible response), call crisis benefits or go to the closest trauma center right away.

* Contact Your Medical Care Supplier: Subsequent to looking for guaranteed clinical consideration, illuminate your medical services supplier about the hypersensitive response. Your medical care supplier will keep the episode in your clinical history and

furnish you with direction on the most proficient method to deal with any future therapy or medicine choices.

* Follow Up: Subsequent to getting crisis treatment, circle back to your medical care supplier for additional assessment and to examine elective therapy choices, if vital. They can assist with distinguishing the particular allergen causing the response and guide you on possible other options.

Recall that hypersensitive responses can be unusual, and it's fundamental for be wary while utilizing any new prescription, including acyclovir. In the event that you have a known sensitivity to acyclovir or any comparative antiviral drug, illuminate your medical care supplier prior to beginning therapy.

* Continuously read the item marking and bundle embed for any medicine you use, and know about the indications of a hypersensitive response. Assuming you experience any surprising side, effects or have worries about the utilization of acyclovir, look for clinical guidance immediately. Early mediation is urgent in overseeing

hypersensitive responses successfully.

CHAPTER FIVE

COLLABORATIONS WITH DIFFERENT DRUGS

Acyclovir can collaborate with different drugs, possibly influencing their adequacy or expanding the gamble of aftereffects. It's critical to illuminate your medical services supplier pretty much every one of the prescriptions, enhancements, and natural items you are taking prior to beginning acyclovir therapy. Here are a few normal collaborations:

* Probenecid: Probenecid is a medicine used to treat gout. It can dial back the disposal of acyclovir from the body, prompting more elevated levels of acyclovir in the circulation system. Assuming that you are taking probenecid, your medical care supplier might have to change the portion of acyclovir to forestall the gamble of harmfulness.

* Nephrotoxic Medications: Acyclovir is essentially killed through the kidneys. Simultaneous utilization of nephrotoxic medications, like specific anti-infection agents (e.g., aminoglycosides) or nonsteroidal calming drugs (NSAIDs), may expand the gamble of kidney harm. Assuming you are taking any nephrotoxic meds, your medical services supplier might have to screen your kidney capability intently while on acyclovir.

* Zidovudine (AZT): Zidovudine is an antiretroviral medicine used to treat HIV. Acyclovir can lessen the

freedom of zidovudine, prompting expanded degrees of zidovudine in the circulation system. Your medical services supplier might have to change the portion of zidovudine assuming that you are taking it alongside acyclovir.

* Interferon: Interferon is utilized to deal with specific viral contaminations and conditions like hepatitis. There have been reports of collaborations among acyclovir and interferon, bringing about an expanded gamble of neurological secondary effects. Your medical services supplier might screen you intently

assuming that you are utilizing these meds together.

* Immunizations: Acyclovir might lessen the adequacy of live antibodies, like the varicella-zoster immunization or the herpes zoster antibody. On the off chance that you are planned to get an immunization, examine with your medical care supplier whether it is protected to get while utilizing acyclovir.

* Other Antiviral Drugs: Taking various antiviral prescriptions together may build the gamble of secondary effects. Assuming you are utilizing other antiviral

medications, your medical services supplier will cautiously survey the expected dangers and advantages prior to endorsing acyclovir.

WELLBEING AND SAFEGUARDS

Security and precautionary measures are significant angles to consider while utilizing acyclovir to guarantee its viability and limit expected gambles. Here are key security measures and safeguards to remember:

* Sensitivities and Touchiness: Illuminate your medical services supplier on the off chance that you have a known sensitivity to

acyclovir or some other antiviral drugs.

On the off chance that you experience indications of a hypersensitive response, like hives, tingling, expanding, or trouble breathing, end the utilization of acyclovir and look for guaranteed clinical consideration.

* Clinical History: Illuminate your medical services supplier about your total clinical history, including any kidney issues, liver issues, or resistant framework problems.

Unveil some other prescriptions, enhancements, or natural items you are taking, as they might communicate with acyclovir.

* Pregnancy and Breastfeeding:

Assuming you are pregnant or intending to become pregnant, talk about the expected dangers and advantages of utilizing acyclovir with your medical services supplier. Acyclovir is by and large thought to be protected during pregnancy when the advantages offset the dangers.

In the event that you are breastfeeding, counsel your medical care supplier prior to utilizing acyclovir, as the medication might be discharged in bosom milk.

* Kidney Capability:

Acyclovir is principally killed through the kidneys. In the event that you have kidney issues or a past filled with kidney sickness, your medical care supplier might change the measurements of acyclovir to forestall potential kidney-related secondary effects.

Remain very much hydrated during acyclovir treatment to help kidney capability, except if prompted in any case by your medical services supplier.

* Drug Connections:

Illuminate your medical services supplier pretty much every one of the meds you are taking, including remedy, non-prescription medications, enhancements, and natural items. Certain meds can collaborate with acyclovir, influencing its viability or expanding the gamble of aftereffects.

* Safe Use in Youngsters: Acyclovir is for the most part ok for use in kids however ought to be utilized under the management of a medical services supplier, particularly in more youthful

youngsters or those with explicit ailments.

* Trying not to Spread the Infection:

To forestall the spread of herpes diseases, try not to contact the mouth blisters or impacted regions pointlessly.

* Clean up completely when applying acyclovir cream.

* Consummation of Treatment:

Follow through with the full endorsed course of acyclovir treatment, regardless of whether your side effects get to the next level. Halting the treatment rashly may prompt deficient goal of the disease.

* Driving and Working Hardware:

Acyclovir isn't known to cause sluggishness or disable mental capacities essentially. In any case, individual reactions might shift. Assuming you experience discombobulation or any unfavorable impacts that might influence your capacity to drive or work apparatus, keep away from such exercises until you feel completely ready.

* Capacity and Removal:

Store acyclovir cream and different details as taught on the bundling. Get it far from youngsters and pets.

Discard any lapsed or unused medicine appropriately, adhering to nearby rules for drug removal.

OUTLINE AND IMPORTANT POINTS ABOUT ACYCLOVIR CREAM

Acyclovir cream is a skin antiviral medicine used to treat viral skin diseases brought about by the herpes simplex infection (HSV), basically HSV-1 (mouth blisters) and HSV-2 (genital herpes), as well as other restricted herpes contaminations. The cream contains acyclovir as its dynamic fixing, which lessens the seriousness of side effects, advance quicker mending, and oversee flare-ups of these viral diseases.

* Rundown of Acyclovir Cream:

Acyclovir cream is utilized to treat mouth blisters (herpes labialis) and outer sores of genital herpes brought about by HSV-1 and HSV-2, individually.

It is additionally successful in dealing with other limited herpes diseases like herpes gladiatorum, herpes whitlow, and herpes simplex keratitis.

CONCLUSION

The cream is applied straightforwardly to the impacted skin surfaces and is best when begun ahead of schedule during the beginning of side effects.

The ordinary dosing is applying the cream like clockwork, five times each day, for a sum of five days.

Acyclovir cream oversees side effects, like agony, tingling, and redness, however doesn't fix herpes diseases or forestall transmission to other people.

The cream is by and large safe for use in many people, yet some might encounter gentle secondary effects like skin aggravation or dryness.

Serious secondary effects are interesting however can incorporate extreme skin responses, hypersensitive responses, and neurological side effects. Look for guaranteed clinical consideration if any of these happen.

* Key Focus points:

Acyclovir cream is a skin antiviral used to treat herpes simplex infection (HSV) contaminations, including mouth blisters and genital herpes, as well as other limited herpes diseases.

It ought to be applied right on time during the beginning of side effects and utilized for the full endorsed course to accomplish the best outcomes.

Assuming you suspect a hypersensitive response or experience extreme aftereffects, look for guaranteed clinical consideration.

Illuminate your medical services supplier about your clinical history and all drugs you are requiring to keep away from expected collaborations or antagonistic impacts.

THE END

Made in United States
Troutdale, OR
10/27/2023

14060224R00040